The Patient's Guide
Ultrasound

ADAM E. M. ELTORAI
DOUGLAS T. HIDLAY
TERRANCE T. HEALEY

Praeclarus Press, LLC
©2019 Douglas T. Hidlay. All rights reserved.

www.PraeclarusPress.com

Praeclarus Press, LLC
2504 Sweetgum Lane
Amarillo, Texas 79124 USA
806-367-9950
www.PraeclarusPress.com

DISCLAIMER
The information contained in this publication is advisory only and
is not intended to replace sound clinical judgment or individualized
patient care. The author disclaims all warranties, whether expressed
or implied, including any warranty as the quality, accuracy, safety,
or suitability of this information for any particular purpose.

ISBN: 978-1-946665-23-2
©2019 Douglas T. Hidlay. All rights reserved.
Email: dhidlayjr@gmail.com

Cover Design: Ken Tackett
Developmental Editing: Kathleen Kendall-Tackett
Copy Editing: Chris Tackett
Layout & Design: Nelly Murariu

CONT

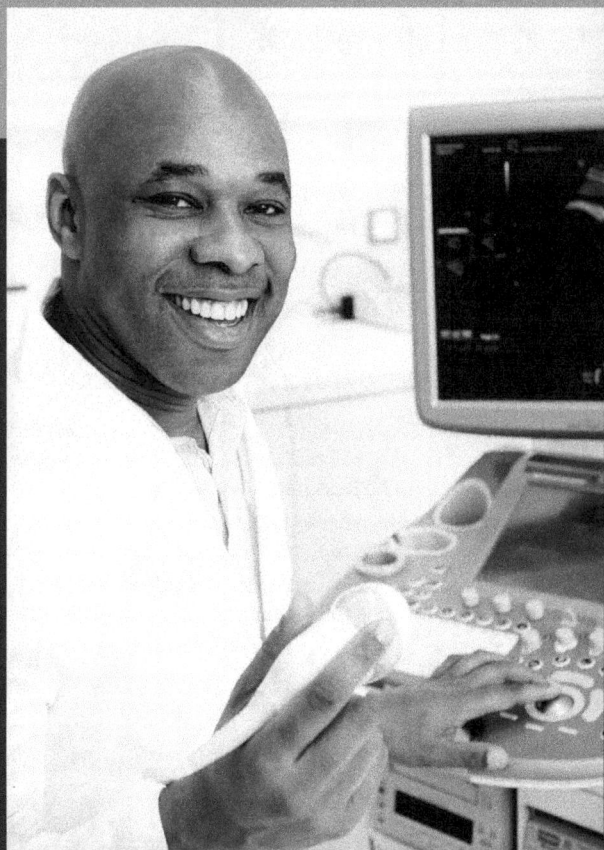

WHAT IS ULTRASOUND?

Ultrasound is a technique that sends sound waves to bounce off an object. A computer then interprets the sound that bounces back to create a picture. In medicine, this allows us to examine various parts of the human body and look for signs of disease. The process is quick, safe, and extremely effective when used to look for the right problem in the right patient.

The term "ultrasound" may also refer to the examination or scan. Scanning is typically performed by a licensed sonographer, someone who is specifically trained in performing this test. Sometimes, it may also be performed by doctors, nurses, or other medical professionals.

The ultrasound machine is made up of a computer, a screen, and a transducer or probe, that transmits the sound waves into the patient. To help the sound waves transmit well, a small amount of gel is often used on the skin over the area to be scanned.

The sound waves used for ultrasound are much higher in frequency, or pitch, than humans or animals can hear. These sound waves travel from the probe through the patient by causing tiny vibrations in the tissues, which are too small to feel. As the tissues vibrate, some of the sound bounces back to the probe. A computer detects this and produces a two-dimensional image on the monitor based on how quickly it hears the echo and

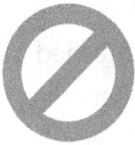

Unlike X-rays or a CAT scan, ultrasound does not use any radiation.

how loud that echo is. Harder structures, like bones, are louder, which is referred to as more echogenic, and the computer displays this as bright on the screen. Things such as fluid do not reflect much sound back, and show up very faintly or not at all. Each organ and tissue has its own appearance on ultrasound and can be inspected for signs of different illnesses.

Unlike X-rays or a CAT scan, ultrasound does not use any radiation. Additionally, it can look at organs and tissues in real time, while X-rays are a still photograph of a body part.

This means that ultrasound can look at how muscles move, or even how blood is flowingin real time. Sometimes patients will be asked to perform certain actions during the ultrasound scan to help the sonographer get the best picture.

Each ultrasound machine has multiple different probes attached to it. These probes have different features that may make one good for looking at a specific organ or tissue, but not another. The sonographer may only need a single probe to do one kind of study, while others may need to switch between several probes to take all of the pictures necessary.

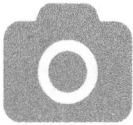

Ultrasound is a painless, noninvasive way of taking pictures inside the human body.

There are many special techniques in ultrasound that can be used in different situations. The machines are capable of taking a short movie clip, or cine, which is useful to record how something is moving. When the test needs to look at blood vessels, a technique known as Doppler might be used, which allows the machine to detect how well and what direction blood is flowing.

In other cases, the machine can be set to create a three-dimensional image instead of the regular 2-D picture. Whether these or other special settings are used varies on a case-by-case basis. Some scans may use none or all of these features as the medical professional decides is needed to make the right diagnosis.

Ultrasound is a painless, noninvasive way of taking pictures inside the human body and is sometimes used to guide a medical procedure. The ultrasound will let the medical professional see the organ or area of interest, and place a needle or other medical instrument in a very precise location in a safe and controlled manner. This is most commonly done to let a needle take a small piece of a tissue, called a biopsy. Other times, ultrasound might be used to place catheters into blood vessels or other parts of the body. If you are getting an ultrasound-guided procedure, additional information about that specific procedure will be provided.

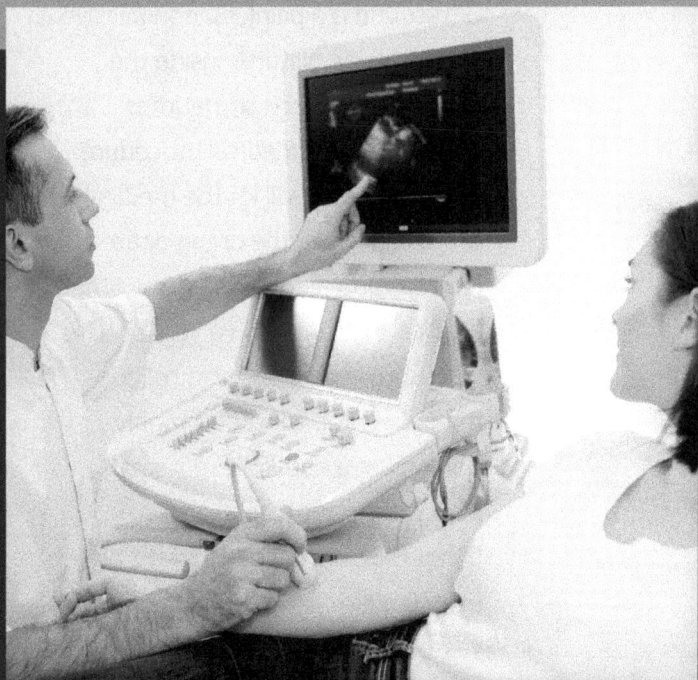

WHY IS ULTRASOUND PERFORMED?

Your provider may order an ultrasound for many different reasons. For one, unlike X-rays or a CAT scan, ultrasound does not use any radiation, so there is not risk associated with performing multiple scans. Ultrasound is very useful for looking at skin, muscle, and blood vessels, as well as the neck, abdomen, pelvis, and heart. Ultrasound is not often ordered for evaluation of the intestines, lungs, or brain.

COMMON REASONS FOR GETTING AN ULTRASOUND

Below is a list of common reasons to get an ultrasound, though certainly not all possible reasons or conditions are covered:

ABDOMINAL ULTRASOUND

To examine the kidneys, liver, gallbladder, spleen pancreas, and abdominal blood vessels

PELVIC ULTRASOUND

To examine the uterus, ovaries, possible pregnancy, and pelvic blood vessels

NECK ULTRASOUND

To examine the thyroid gland, lymph nodes, salivary glands, and neck blood vessels

MUSCULOSKELETAL ULTRASOUND

To examine muscles, tendons, and ligaments

DEDICATED VASCULAR ULTRASOUND

To examine the arteries and/or veins of one or multiple extremities

Sometimes these scans are looking to answer a specific question, such as "are there gallstones?" or "is there a thyroid nodule?" Other times, they are ordered to look more generally for a problem in part of the body.

Based on the information and concerns of the ordering clinician, the scans will be adjusted and targeted to answer the questions specific to your signs or symptoms.

It can be very helpful for the sonographer or clinician who is performing your ultrasound to know certain information that may help them guide your scan.

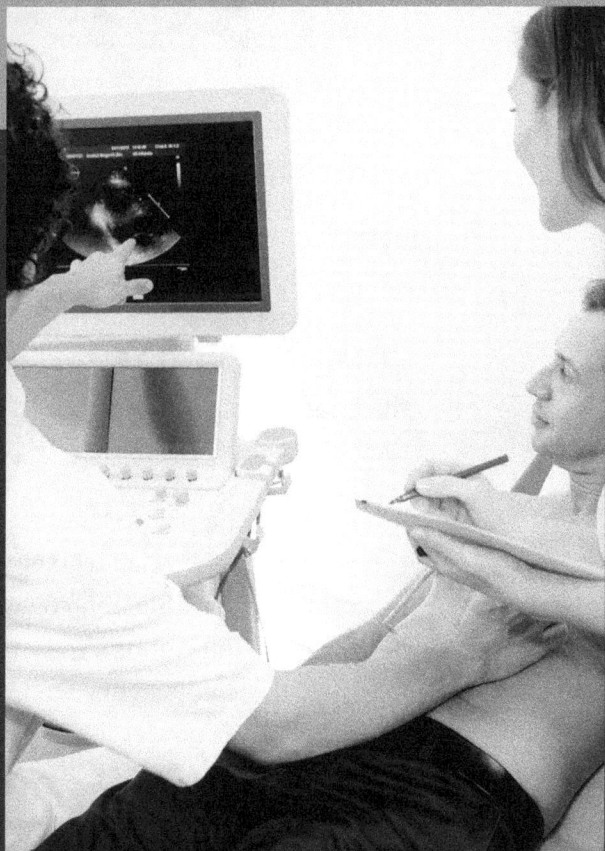

HOW DO I PREPARE FOR MY ULTRASOUND?

The specific preparation for an ultrasound varies based on what body part will be scanned and what questions are trying to be answered. Below, general guidelines for preparing for an ultrasound are given by body part. For many scans, you will need to do little advanced preparation before the exam. Any specific preparation for your scan should be provided to you ahead of time. In most cases, you will be asked to change into a hospital gown. This will be helpful for the sonographer but also protect your clothes from getting any ultrasound gel on them.

Abdominal Ultrasound

Most abdominal ultrasounds are performed with a patient fasting, or NPO, for six or eight hours ahead of time. This minimizes how much gas is in the intestines, which could obscure organs and limit the study. Fasting is especially important when evaluating the structure of the right upper abdomen; specifically, the liver and gallbladder. Eating before a scan of these organs may limit the ability to diagnose some conditions and require more testing.

If the ultrasound will focus on the kidneys, you may be asked to drink several glasses of water in the hour or two before a study to keep you hydrated and help ensure an adequate look at the kidneys and bladder. Any medications you normally take can still be taken with a small sip of water at their regular time.

Pelvic Ultrasound

Most pelvic ultrasounds are performed after having a patient drink 32 ounces of water an hour ahead of time and doing their best to not urinate during that time. This allows the sonographer the best window to look at the uterus and ovaries. If you feel you cannot wait this long without using the restroom, please let your sonographer know. Otherwise, you may eat and drink normally in the time leading up to the scan. Any medications you normally take can still be taken at their regular time.

Neck, Musculoskeletal, and Vascular Ultrasound

These tests do not routinely require any special preparation in advance. You may eat and drink normally ahead of time and take any medications as usual.

WHAT IS THE EQUIPMENT LIKE?

An ultrasound machine is composed of three main components. The probe, or transducer, is connected to the machine by a typical computer cable. This part sends out the ultrasound waves and listens for them to bounce back. These will vary in size and shape based on their function.

The signals these detect are sent to the ultrasound machine, which is a specialized computer with a control panel, and the picture is displayed on a high definition monitor, not unlike a many computer screens.

WHAT DOES THE PROCEDURE INVOLVE?

Ultrasound scans are safe and noninvasive. In most cases, you will be asked to change into a hospital gown before the exam begins. You will be taken to a small, quiet room, where your scan can be performed privately. If you would like a family member or friend to accompany you, you can do so for most studies.

Each type of scan requires its own specific positioning and takes a different amount of time. The sonographer will guide you through any movements or actions they may need you to perform. The better you are able to follow his or her instructions, the quicker and more thorough examination they can perform.

A small amount of gel will be applied to your skin to help the ultrasound take better pictures and may need to be reapplied during the exam. You will feel some pressure as the ultrasound is directed over various parts of the body. If this becomes uncomfortable, please let the sonographer know. There is rarely any other source of discomfort during the test. At the end of the scan, any left over gel will be cleaned off your skin.

Abdominal Ultrasound

These scans tend to take longer than other examinations, but not always. Much of the scanning can be done while lying flat on your back. Often times, you will be asked to hold your breath to look in the upper abdomen for 10 to 20 seconds at a time. You

will often need to take turns rolling
onto your sides for part of the scan.
You may be asked to drink water
if the scan involves looking at the
kidneys and bladder.

Pelvic Ultrasound

These scans may be done in one or
two parts and tend to take less than
an hour. Most of the scanning will
be done with you lying on your back.
The first portion of the exam will be
done transabdominally, by scanning
from your belly to look down through
the full bladder at the uterus and
ovaries.

The second portion of the exam,
if necessary, will be performed
transvaginally, by using a special
small probe to look at the uterus and
ovaries through the vagina. This may
be uncomfortable but is the best way
to look at the uterus and ovaries for
signs of disease in most cases. If you

have never been sexually active, please let the sonographer know as the transvaginal examination can be omitted in some cases.

If you have any pain or discomfort during the exam, it is important to tell the sonographer, as this can be helpful in making the correct diagnosis.

Neck, Musculoskeletal, and Vascular Ultrasound

These scans tend to be done in less than an hour. Most of the scanning will be done with you lying on your back, though you may be asked to move or turn for some portions of the exam. It is likely that the sonographer will instruct you to perform certain motions or need to move you to help their exam. If you have any pain or discomfort during the exam, it is important to tell the sonographer, as this can be helpful in making the correct diagnosis.

WHAT DOES AN ULTRASOUND SCAN FEEL LIKE?

Ultrasound scans are safe and noninvasive. The only sensation that may be unpleasant for most people during an exam comes from the pressure of the probe on the skin.

The sonographer may need to push quite firmly on your skin and tissues to visualize certain structures. If this becomes too unpleasant, it is important to let them know.

After the ultrasound is done, you should have no residual discomfort or symptoms.

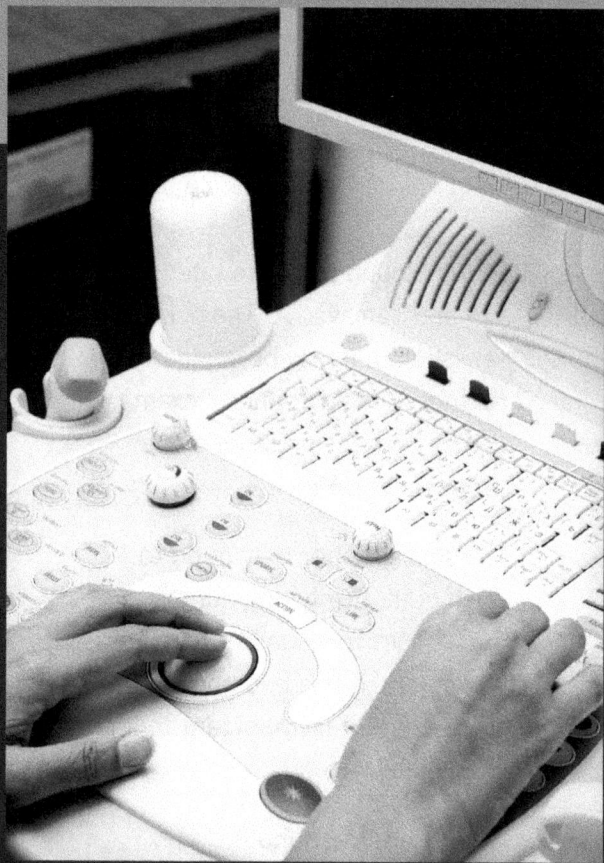

WHAT HAPPENS AFTER THE PROCEDURE?

After the ultrasound procedure is done, you will be allowed to go home and carry on about your day as usual, in most cases.

There are no restrictions or special instructions after someone has an ultrasound, unless there was something seen that would need immediate attention or specific care. If that were the case, a practitioner would immediately come let you know and speak to the doctor or clinician who referred you for the scan.

If you have questions during or after the scan, you may be able to have them answered right then and there. Let your sonographer know your concerns and a clinician may be able to discuss them with you during or after the ultrasound.

How Will I Know The Results Of My Scan?

Once your scan is finished, a sonographer will review the images with a doctor specialized in that test, usually a Radiologist. He or she will look at the images and send a report to your health care provider who asked for the ultrasound. Your provider will either call you or have you come in to be seen to discuss the results, typically within a week.

In some cases, a Radiologist can give you the results of the test right then. Other times, they need to review the case and discuss it with your doctor before the results will be available. If your results are not immediately available, it does not mean that something concerning was found; rather, it may be that the radiologist and your provider want to come up with a plan to find an explanation for your symptoms because the study was normal.

If you have questions or concerns, please let your sonographer know and someone should be available to talk to you.

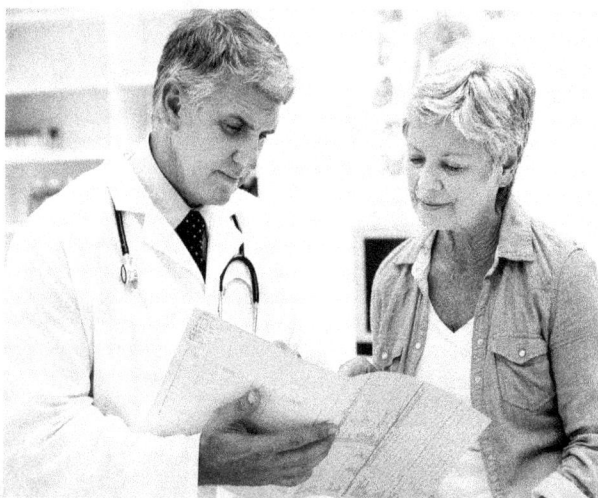

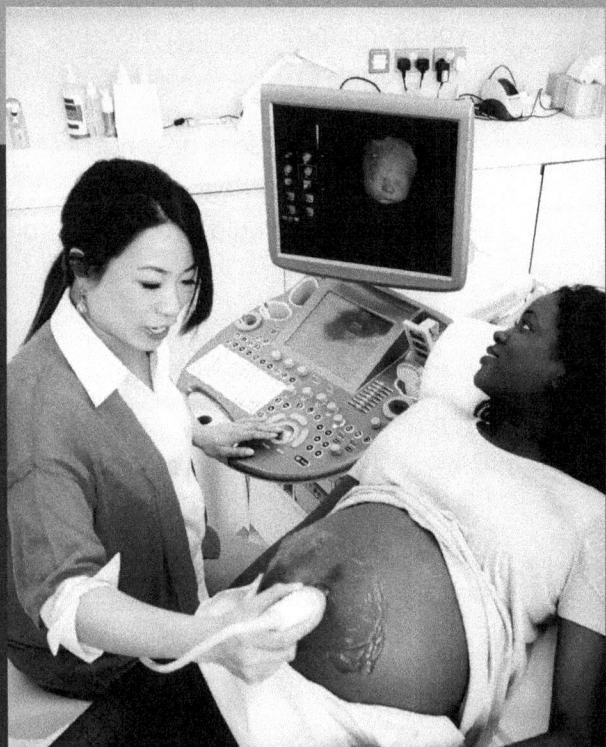

WHAT ARE THE RISKS OF ULTRASOUND? WHAT ARE THE BENEFITS?

Ultrasound is extremely safe and effective. There has never been a single documented case of injury or illness caused by medical ultrasound since it was first used in 1956. That said, there are theoretical risks to ultrasound and certain precautions are taken for sake of prudence. The two things that are monitored and kept as low as possible are the thermal index and the mechanical index. These are measures of how the ultrasound waves may affect the tissues.

When the ultrasound wave goes through a tissue, it causes tiny vibrations. Some of this energy becomes heat in those tissues. The thermal index is a way to measure how much heat could be made by the ultrasound waves. This number is kept below certain limits to make sure no significant heating occurs. Certain techniques, like Doppler, could deposit more heat than typical ultrasound. This is also monitored as a precautionary measure.

The mechanical index refers to how much vibration the ultrasound waves causes in the tissues they pass through. At normal levels, these vibrations are virtually imperceptible to patients. In some specific cases, the ultrasound settings may be changed intentionally to cause more vibration. If your exam might involve this, you would

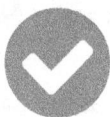

The benefits of ultrasound are significant.

be told ahead of time that you might feel the vibrations faintly at certain points. Again, these tiny vibrations have never been shown to cause harm to any human in more than 70 years of use.

The benefits of ultrasound are significant.

Are There Limitations to Ultrasound?

Ultrasound is very effective test for many different medical conditions, but it is not perfect by any means. The primary limitations relate to resolution, power, and artifacts. These will affect what can be seen, how well things can be seen, and how clearly the images can be interpreted.

Resolution is a measure of how well small details can be seen using a particular probe.

This is primarily related to the pitch of the ultrasound waves, also known as its frequency. Higher frequencies are able to distinguish very small details well, but they are not able to send ultrasound waves through harder structures. Lower frequencies will miss these small details but are able to look at a larger amount of tissue at a time.

Power refers to how far the ultrasound waves can travel before they are too weak to bounce back. Lower frequency probes have more power and can see deeper into a person but have worse resolution. Higher frequency probes are able to make out more details, but their sound waves are weaker and the can only see a much shallower depth. This can be a particular issue as patients get larger and may limit how confident a diagnosis can be made.

The last common issue that may limit an ultrasound scan is the presence of certain artifacts, which are when the computer incorrectly interprets the sound waves that are bouncing back. Believe it or not, certain artifacts are very helpful to making the right diagnosis. A cyst, which is a benign fluid-filled structure common in the liver or kidneys, tricks the computer into thinking all the tissue behind it is more echogenic, or brighter, than it should be. This can be a very important sign that there is nothing to worry about.

Other artifacts are much more problematic, most commonly shadowing. Shadowing is when a structure is so hard that it doesn't let any sound pass through. The computer will struggle to see through bones, gas, and sometimes even certain organs, which means the areas behind these tissues cannot be seen.

Many times, the sonographer can reposition and look around the area from a different spot, but sometimes parts of the body simply cannot be seen. When this happens, your provider may need to order a second test if that is part of why he or she wanted the ultrasound.

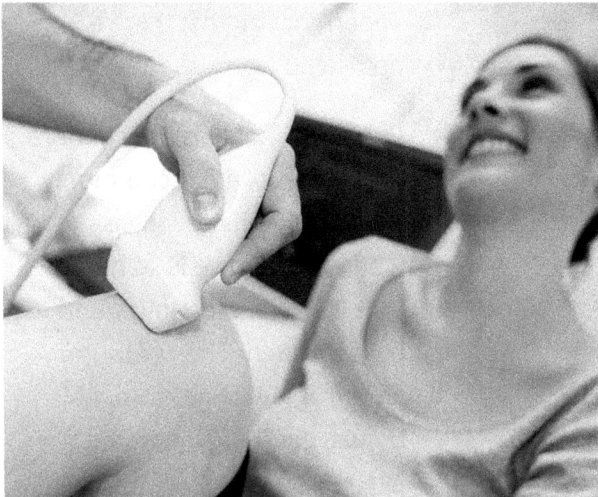

FREQUENTLY ASKED QUESTIONS

Does ultrasound involve any radiation?

No. Ultrasound uses sound waves to create a picture.

Are there any risks to an ultrasound?

While there are theoretical risks, no injury has ever been documented in a patient due to an ultrasound scan.

How long will my ultrasound take?

It varies based on the study but usually less than an hour for a test.

When will my results be available?

It varies based on the study, but you should have results within a week.

GLOSSARY

ARTIFACTS

Errors in the computer interpreting the returning ultrasound waves.

BIOPSY

A procedure where a small piece of a tissue is taken for evaluation by a laboratory and under a microscope.

CINE

A short movie of ultrasound images.

DOPPLER

A special technique that can detect flowing blood or fluid.

ECHO

The reflection of ultrasound waves off a tissue or organ.

ECHOGENIC

An adjective used to describe how bright or dark something is on ultrasound. A bright object is "hyperechoic," while a dark one is "hypoechoic."

MECHANICAL INDEX

A measurement of how strong the vibrations are during a scan.

NPO

A Latin term used in medicine, which is short for *nils per os*, which means "nothing by mouth."

RESOLUTION

The ability for the computer to make out small details.

POWER

How far the ultrasound waves can go before they are too weak to bounce back.

PROBE

A shorthand way of referring to the transducer, which emits and receives the ultrasound waves.

SCAN

A shorthand way of referring to an ultrasound examination

SHADOWING

When sound waves cannot see behind a
structure and everything appears dark.

SONOGRAPHER

A medical professional licensed
and trained to perform ultrasound
examinations.

THERMAL INDEX

A measurement of how much heat a
scan is generating.

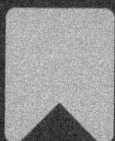

ADDITIONAL RESOURCES

www.rsna.org

www.acr.org

www.nibib.nih.gov

www.mayoclinic.org

MY CONTACTS

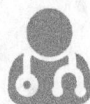

NAME

CONTACT

NAME

CONTACT

NAME

CONTACT

NAME

CONTACT

MY APPOINTMENTS

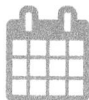

MONDAY

Date:
_____

TUESDAY

Date:
_____

WEDNESDAY

Date:
_____

THURSDAY

Date:
_____

FRIDAY

Date:
_____

SATURDAY

Date:
_____

MY QUESTIONS

MY QUESTIONS

MY NOTES

MY NOTES

MY NOTES